THE DANGERS OF DRUGS, ALCOHOL, AND SMOKING

THE DANGERS OF
PRESCRIPTION DRUGS

KRISTIN THIEL

PowerKiDS
press
New York

Published in 2020 by The Rosen Publishing Group, Inc.
29 East 21st Street, New York, NY 10010

First Edition

Editor: Jenna Tolli
Book Design: Reann Nye

Photo Credits: Cover Inti St Clair/Getty Images; series art patpitchaya/Shutterstock.com; p. 5 Paul Bradbury/ OJO Images/Getty Images; p. 7 Gligatron/Shutterstock.com; p. 8 Sherry Yates Young/ Shutterstock.com; p. 9 B. Boissonnet/ Corbis Documentary / Getty Images Plus/Getty Images; p. 11 Daily Herald Archive/ SSPL/Getty Images; p. 12 Cherngchay Donkhuntod/Shutterstock.com; pp. 13, 17 Monkey Business Images/Shutterstock.com; p. 15 Tetra Images/Getty Images; p. 16 stefanel/Shutterstock. com; p. 19 Photographee.eu/Shutterstock.com; p. 21 Feng Yu/Shutterstock.com; p. 22 Andrey_Popov/ Shutterstock.com.

Cataloging-in-Publication Data

Names: Thiel, Kristin.
Title: The dangers of prescription drugs / Kristin Thiel.
Description: New York : PowerKids Press, 2020. | Series: The dangers of drugs, alcohol, and smoking | Includes glossary and index.
Identifiers: ISBN 9781725309869 (pbk.) | ISBN 9781725309883 (library bound) | ISBN 9781725309876 (6 pack)
Subjects: LCSH: Medication abuse–Juvenile literature. | Drug abuse–Juvenile literature.
Classification: LCC HV5809.5 T57 2020 | DDC 362.299–dc23

Manufactured in the United States of America

Some of the images in this book illustrate individuals who are models. The depictions do not imply actual situations or events.

CPSIA Compliance Information: Batch #CWPK20. For Further Information contact Rosen Publishing, New York, New York at 1-800-237-9932.

CONTENTS

THE POWER OF PRESCRIPTION DRUGS

When you're sick or if you get hurt, your parent or guardian might give you medicine to help you feel better. Sometimes, your doctor might ask you to take **prescription** drugs. Doctors prescribe, or officially recommend, that people use prescription drugs to help them with certain medical problems.

Prescription drugs can help you get healthy, but you have to be careful when you use them. They can be very dangerous, or unsafe, if you use them in the wrong way or if you don't follow the directions. Understanding how prescription drugs work and how to use them correctly can help you stay safe.

DANGER ZONE

There are differences between prescription drugs and illegal drugs. Prescription drugs are legal and doctors prescribe them to help people feel better. It's never safe to use illegal drugs.

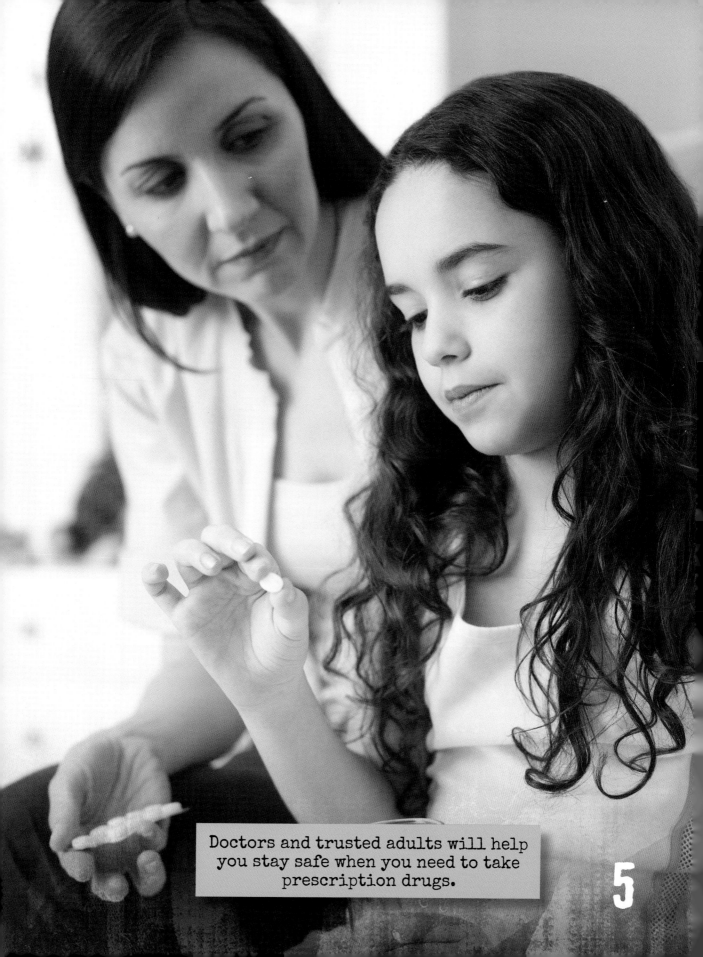

Doctors and trusted adults will help you stay safe when you need to take prescription drugs.

5

PRESCRIPTION DRUGS VS. OTC DRUGS

Different kinds of drugs help to treat different illnesses or medical problems. Some drugs need a prescription from a doctor, but others can be purchased without one. These are called over-the-counter drugs, or OTC drugs. These drugs can be found on the shelf at grocery stores and convenience stores.

OTC drugs are used to treat problems that are minor, or less serious, than ones that need prescriptions. Fevers, colds, and sore throats are common problems that can be solved with OTC drugs. Even though a prescription is not needed, parents should still talk to the doctor to find the right kind of medicine for kids.

DANGER ZONE

In the United States, the Food and Drug Administration (FDA) **regulates** prescription and OTC drugs. The FDA makes sure drugs are safe before they can be used.

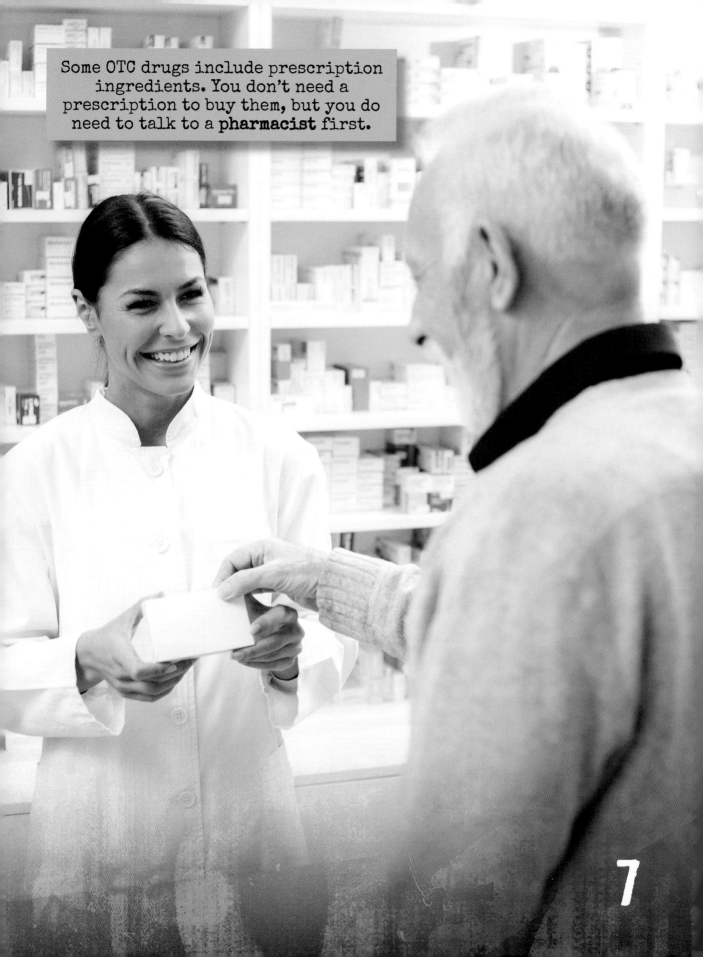

Some OTC drugs include prescription ingredients. You don't need a prescription to buy them, but you do need to talk to a **pharmacist** first.

7

HOW DO THEY WORK?

Prescription drugs need to travel through your body to do their job. Medicine enters your body when you swallow a pill or liquid, or when you get a shot. Then, your blood carries most drugs through your body to the place where they are needed. After the medicine has helped you, your body breaks it down.

DANGER ZONE

Antibiotics are prescription drugs that can help cure some types of **infections**. They have helped millions of people, but they don't work as well when they're used too much.

Rx Pha

AMOXICILLIN 500 MG

TAKE ONE CAPSULE B
MOUTH 2X PER DAY F
DAYS

QTY: 20

No Refills. Dr. Auth Required

ed: 12-01-2016

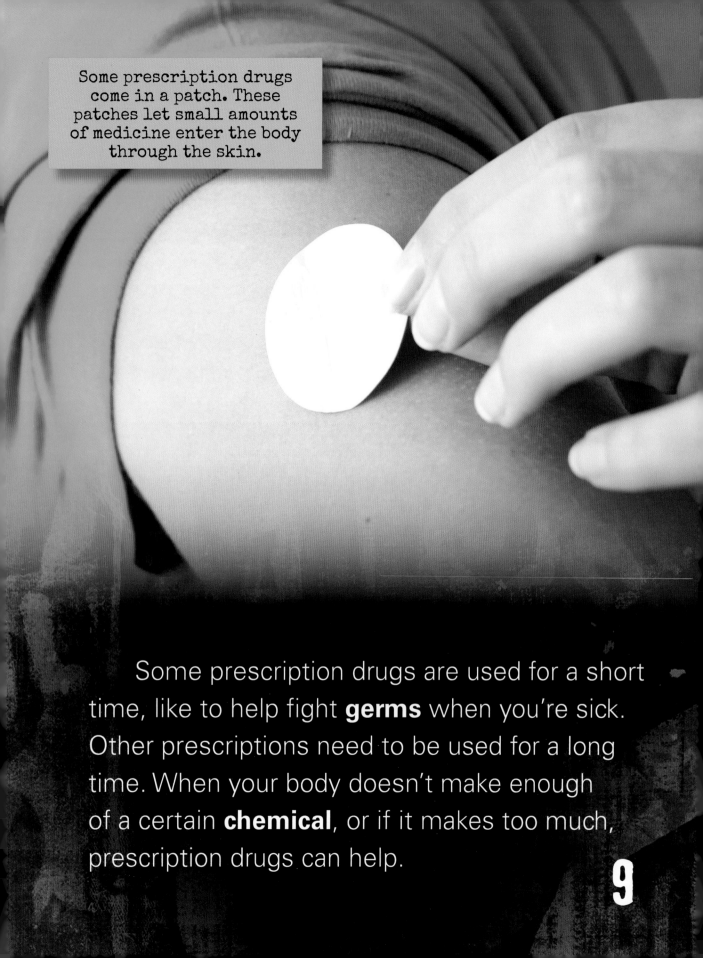

Some prescription drugs come in a patch. These patches let small amounts of medicine enter the body through the skin.

Some prescription drugs are used for a short time, like to help fight **germs** when you're sick. Other prescriptions need to be used for a long time. When your body doesn't make enough of a certain **chemical**, or if it makes too much, prescription drugs can help.

THE HISTORY OF PAINKILLERS

Opioids are one type of commonly misused prescription drug. Doctors prescribe opioids to patients to help **relieve** their pain. Misusing opioids can lead to opioid **addiction**, which has become a serious public health problem in the United States.

In the 1800s, a pharmacist in Germany used the opium poppy plant to make a painkiller. During the Civil War, doctors in the army gave these painkillers to soldiers. The drug helped a lot of people, but some people also became addicted. Even 150 years ago, doctors were concerned that using opioids could be dangerous.

DANGER ZONE

Every year, almost 12,000 children and teenagers in the United States try opioids that were not prescribed to them. This can lead to serious harm or even death.

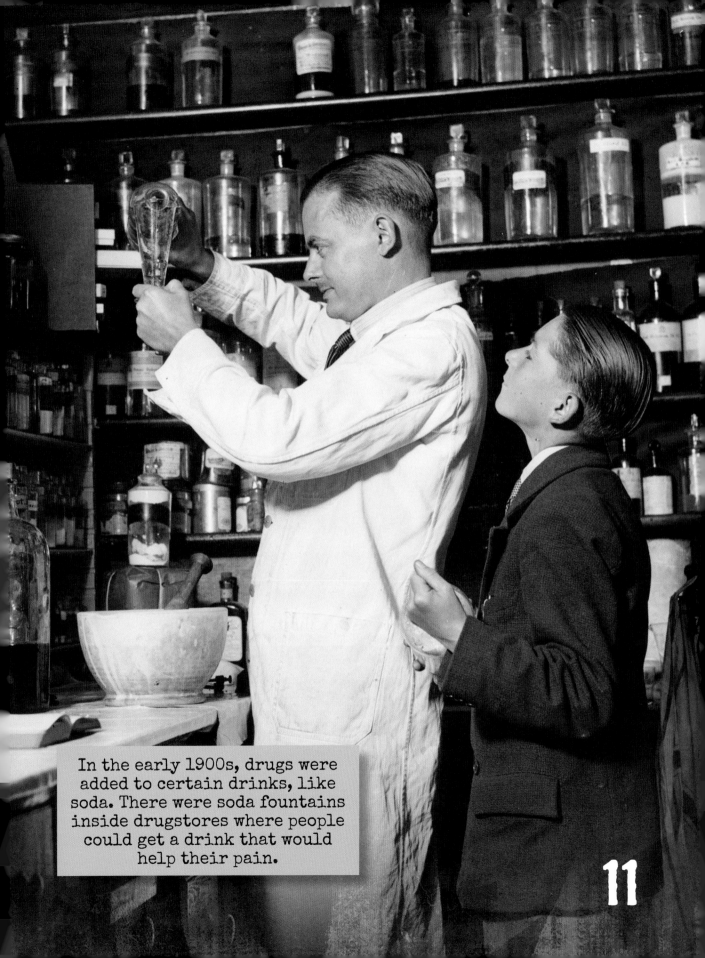

In the early 1900s, drugs were added to certain drinks, like soda. There were soda fountains inside drugstores where people could get a drink that would help their pain.

WARNING! DANGER AHEAD!

Taking any kind of prescription drug is serious. It's important to follow all of the doctor's directions any time you take a prescription drug to make sure you use it safely.

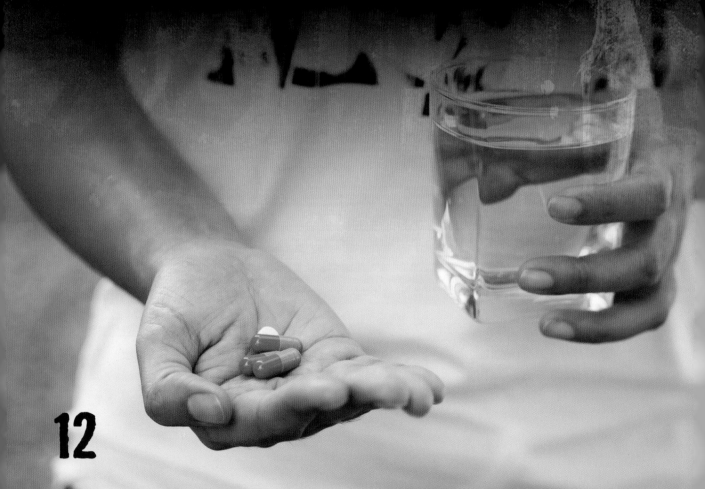

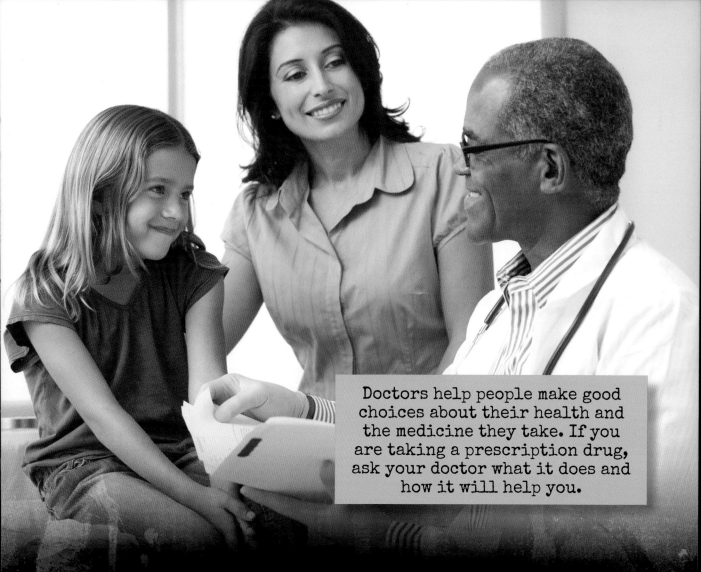

Doctors help people make good choices about their health and the medicine they take. If you are taking a prescription drug, ask your doctor what it does and how it will help you.

For example, you should never take more or less of the drug than what was prescribed. If you don't feel like the drug is working, or if you start to feel different when you use it, make sure you tell your parents and doctor immediately. Your doctor might change the drug you're taking if you have bad **symptoms**, or they might change the **dose** of the drug.

13

EVERYONE IS DIFFERENT

Doctors only give prescription drugs to patients after they have talked to them, and when they know the drug can help with the patient's medical problem. Even if you are having the same problem as a friend or family member, you should never use another person's prescription. Everyone is different! If a drug has not been prescribed for you, it is not safe for you to use.

There might be prescription drugs in your house, but they are against the law to use if they're not yours. It is illegal to use someone else's prescription or to share your own prescriptions with other people.

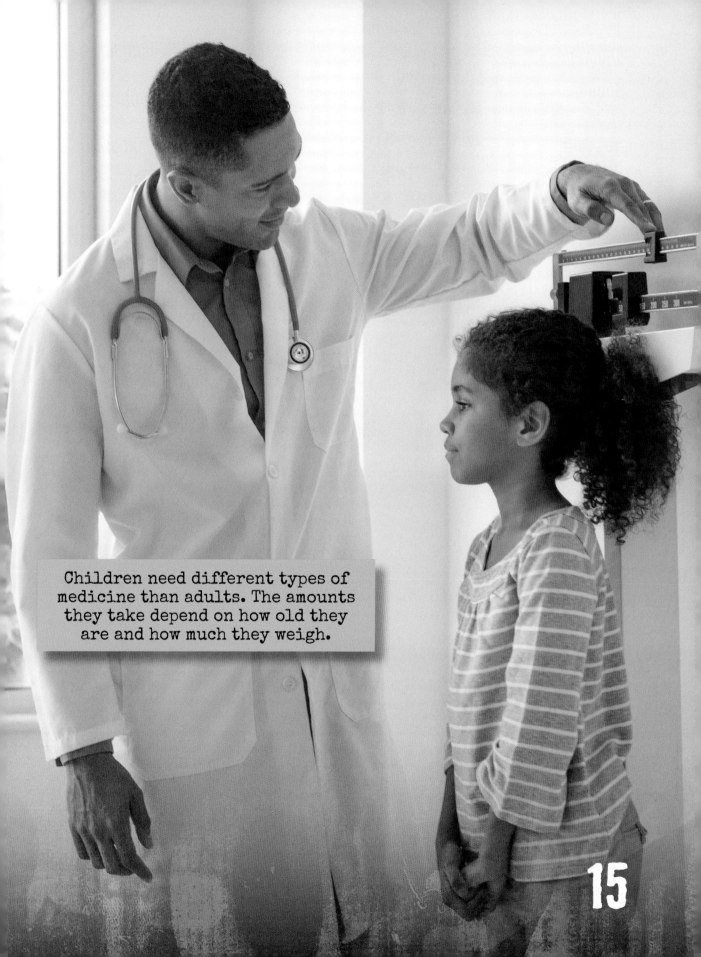

Children need different types of medicine than adults. The amounts they take depend on how old they are and how much they weigh.

15

PRESCRIPTION DRUG ABUSE

Prescription drug abuse is when someone uses drugs in a way that was not approved by their doctor. Using medicine in the wrong way can make you feel sick or confused. It can also make it hard to breathe, or change how fast your heart beats. This can lead to serious illness and even death.

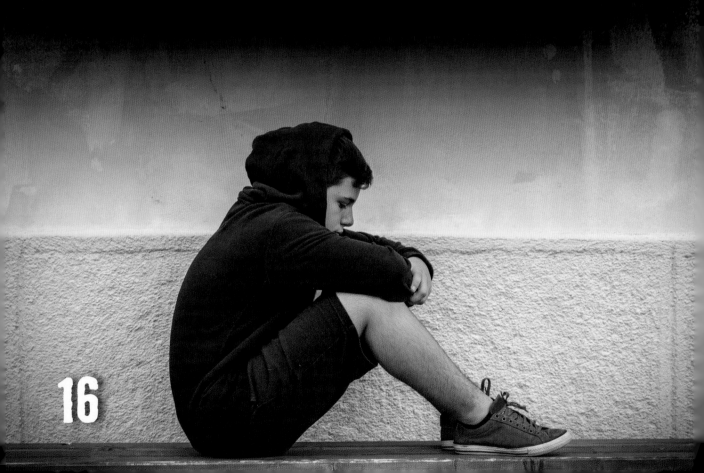

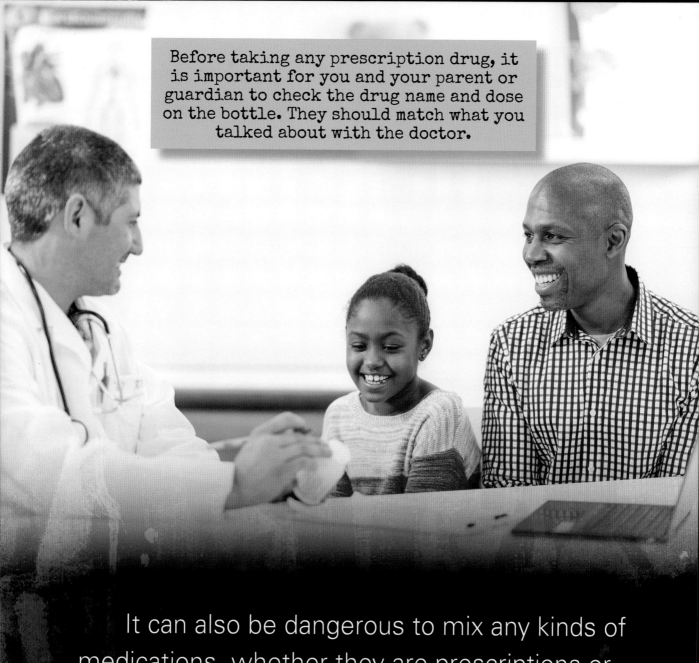

Before taking any prescription drug, it is important for you and your parent or guardian to check the drug name and dose on the bottle. They should match what you talked about with the doctor.

It can also be dangerous to mix any kinds of medications, whether they are prescriptions or over-the-counter drugs. Using certain drugs at the same time can raise the risk of serious health problems, like heart failure. It's always important to talk to your parents and your doctor before you take any kind of medication.

HOW TO HELP

Using prescription drugs the wrong way can cause bad side effects, but it can also lead to addiction. When someone is addicted to a drug, they feel like they always need to have it. When someone is using prescription drugs, they should check in with their doctor regularly. Doctors observe their patients to make sure the drug is working and that they are not becoming addicted.

If you are worried about someone who is using prescription drugs, or if you notice that someone has been giving their prescription drugs to others, talk to your parents or a teacher. They will be able to find help.

DANGER ZONE

It can be very hard for people to stop taking a drug if they are addicted to it. They might keep using the drug even if it is causing problems.

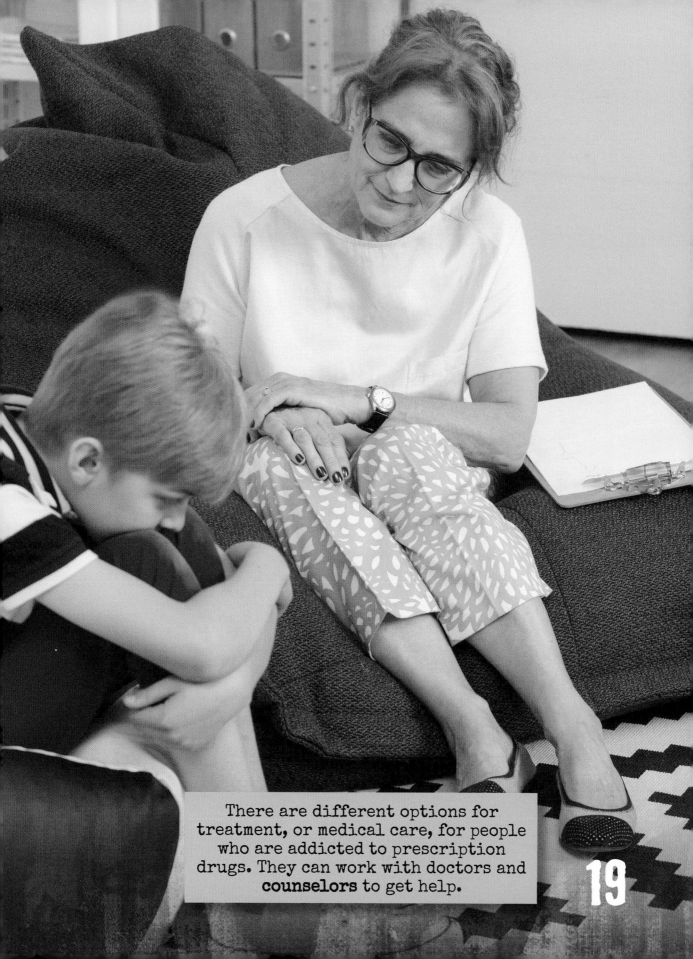

There are different options for treatment, or medical care, for people who are addicted to prescription drugs. They can work with doctors and **counselors** to get help.

You can stay safe when using prescription drugs by learning more about them and being careful any time you use them. Always ask an adult to help when you need to take them. Never offer your prescription drugs to other people, and never take a drug that was prescribed to someone else.

When you are hurt or sick, always be honest with your doctor about what you feel. This will help them know what kind of medicine is best for you. Make sure you tell them about any medicine you have taken recently too. Many drugs do not work well together and can be even more dangerous.

DANGER ZONE

If you have a younger brother or sister, make sure you keep medicine out of their reach. They could take it by mistake, which can be very harmful.

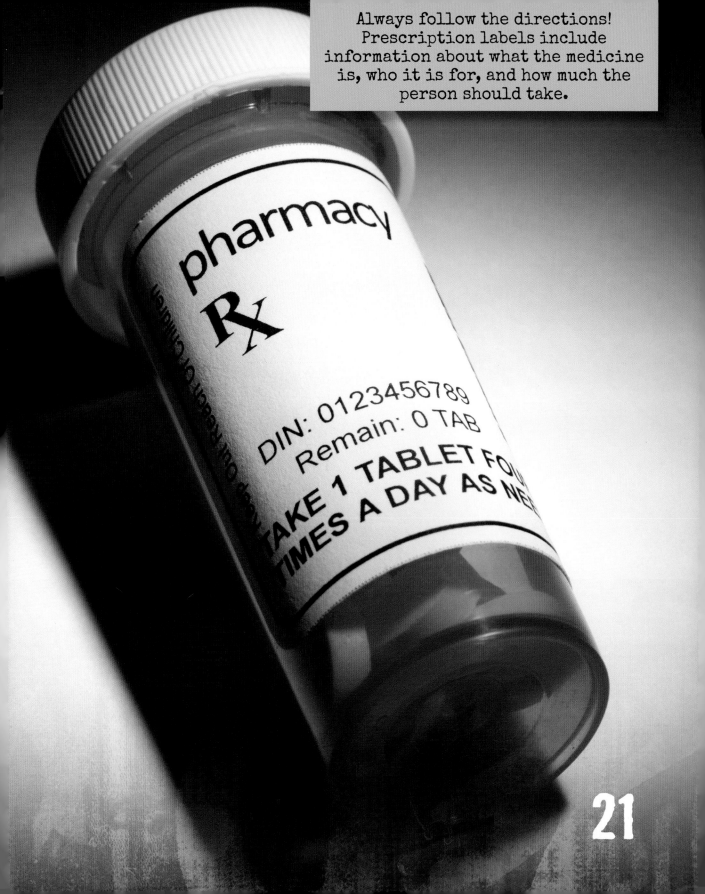

Always follow the directions! Prescription labels include information about what the medicine is, who it is for, and how much the person should take.

pharmacy

Rx

DIN: 0123456789
Remain: 0 TAB

TAKE 1 TABLET FOUR
TIMES A DAY AS NEE

21

STAYING SAFE

Thanks to prescription drugs, many illnesses and medical problems can be treated. There are many benefits to prescription drugs, but they also come with important risks. It is not safe to take a prescription drug that was not prescribed to you, or to take an amount that your doctor didn't approve.

Make sure you always talk to a parent or a guardian about the safety of any medicine you use. When you see drug ads online or on television, ask what they're for and how they work. As you learn more about prescription drugs, you can help teach others how to stay safe, too!

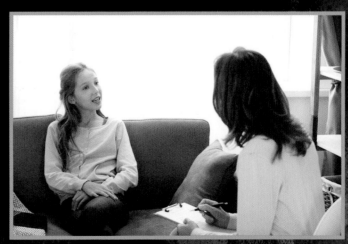

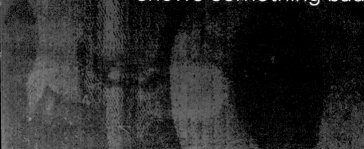

WEBSITES

Due to the changing nature of Internet links, PowerKids Press has developed an online list of websites related to the subject of this book. This site is updated regularly. Please use this link to access the list: www.powerkidslinks.com/das/prescription